EATING ONE MEAL A DAY: The Science and Benefits of OMAD Fasting

By Yuri G Allman

INTRODUCTION

Welcome to "The OMAD Diet: An Introduction to One Meal a Day Fasting for Health and Well-being." In this book, we will explore the world of OMAD (One Meal a Day) fasting, a type of intermittent fasting that involves eating just one meal per day.

Throughout this book, we will delve into the history and science of OMAD fasting, discuss the potential benefits and drawbacks of this dietary pattern, and provide tips and strategies for successfully incorporating OMAD fasting into your routine.

Whether you are new to OMAD fasting or have been practicing it for some time, this book will provide you with the tools you need to optimize your OMAD fasting practice and achieve your health and wellness goals.

We will begin by exploring the history of OMAD fasting and how it fits into the larger context of intermittent fasting. We will then discuss the potential benefits of OMAD fasting and the current state of research on this topic.

Next, we will delve into the practicalities of practicing OMAD fasting, including how to structure your eating window, choose nutrient-dense foods, and manage hunger and cravings. We will also discuss the importance of staying active and maintaining energy while following an OMAD fasting routine.

Finally, we will provide tips and strategies for success with OMAD fasting, including how to handle setbacks and common mistakes to avoid. By the end of this book, you will have a solid foundation in the principles of OMAD fasting and the tools you need to make this dietary pattern work for you.

So, let's get started on your journey to improved health and well-being with OMAD fasting.

CHAPTER 1

Introduction to Intermittent Fasting

Definition and History of Intermittent Fasting

Intermittent fasting: definition and background

A dietary strategy called intermittent fasting includes alternating between fasting and eating intervals. Intermittent fasting comes in a variety of forms, but they all entail limiting food intake for a certain amount of time. The 5:2 diet, which includes eating normally for 5 days and limiting food intake to 500–600 calories for the other 2 days, and the 16/8 approach, which requires fasting for 16 hours and eating within an 8-hour window, are the two most popular types of intermittent fasting.

Ancient civilizations had a long history of intermittent fasting, which was often practiced for religious or spiritual reasons. In more recent times, intermittent fasting has been utilized to enhance health and treat certain medical disorders. In more recent times, intermittent fasting has been utilized to enhance health and treat certain medical disorders. It has gained popularity recently as a method of weight management and for its conceivable health advantages, such as greater weight loss, better insulin sensitivity, and decreased inflammation. It is crucial to remember that more study is required to properly understand the consequences of intermittent fasting and that not everyone is a good candidate for it. Before beginning any new eating pattern, it is usually a good idea to consult with a healthcare provider.

Types of Intermittent Fasting: There are several varieties of intermittent fasting, including the 16/8 strategy, the 5:2 diet, and alternate-day fasting. The 16/8 approach calls for limiting a person's daily meal consumption to an 8-hour window, such as from 12 to 8 p.m., then fasting for the next 16 hours. In the 5:2 diet, you consume normally for five days while limiting your calorie intake to 500–600 for the other two days that are not consecutive. By eating regularly one day and just 500–600 calories the following, you may practice alternate-day fasting.

Although there is little data on the benefits of OMAD fasting, several studies have shown that it may help people lose weight and improve their insulin sensitivity. It is crucial to remember that further study is required in order to completely comprehend the consequences of OMAD fasting and the long-term security of this eating pattern.

Calorie intake: It's critical to ensure that you are obtaining enough calories and nutrients to support your body's demands while on the OMAD diet. This might be difficult since you have to eat all of your daily calorie intake at once. Make sure you are eating meals that are nutrient-dense, rich in protein, fiber, and healthy fats, and that you are receiving enough vitamins and minerals.

Health Benefits: Studies have shown that intermittent fasting may have a number of health advantages, including better insulin sensitivity, decreased inflammation, and weight reduction. Additionally, it could be advantageous for heart health indicators, including blood pressure and cholesterol levels. To completely comprehend the consequences of intermittent fasting and the long-term safety of this eating pattern, further study is necessary; it is vital to emphasize this.

Who Can Benefit: People who are overweight or obese may find intermittent fasting helpful since it can aid in weight reduction and improve insulin sensitivity. While it is critical to consult with a healthcare provider before beginning any new dietary pattern, it may also be beneficial for people who have certain medical conditions, such as type 2 diabetes or high blood pressure. Not everyone should practice intermittent fasting, and those with specific medical issues, pregnant women, or nursing mothers should avoid it.

Potential Risks: In the beginning of intermittent fasting, side symptoms including hunger, irritability, and trouble focusing are possible. During the times when you aren't fasting, it's crucial to consume adequate nutrition and keep hydrated. Medications and nutritional supplements that must be taken with meals may be affected by intermittent fasting as well. Before beginning any new eating pattern, it is usually a good idea to consult with a healthcare provider.

Think about: If you're thinking about attempting the OMAD diet, be sure you're consuming enough calories and nutrients to support your body's demands. Additionally, it's critical to drink enough water and choose meals that are nutrient-dense and rich in protein, fiber, and healthy fats. Before beginning any new eating pattern, it is usually a good idea to consult with a healthcare provider.

What Can Happen if You Eat Only One Meal a Day

A diet consisting mostly of fatty, whole animal meals may have a variety of positive effects when just one meal is consumed each day.

The many advantages of OMAD for health and way of life include:

Streamlining how you feel about food and eating
Making extra time and space in the mind for other pursuits, interactions, development, and professional objectives
Encourage digestion and intestinal health
Encourage the renewal of cells (autophagy)
Reduce your weight.
reduced autoimmune diseases and inflammation

increase sensitivity and balance of hormones
Let's go more deeply into a couple of these
important OMAD results.

Fits Your Current Eating Patterns with
Biological Evolution
Eating just one meal a day contrasts with the
typical American diet, which consists of three
meals and two snacks each day.

Prior to the domestication of plants around
10,000 years ago, when humans had been
evolving for over 2 million years, feasting on
enormous meals and fasting in between was
probably the norm.

This is so because humans were apex predators
who feasted on enormous animals or the spoils
of successful hunts before going without food
until the next hunt. Since there was no
refrigeration, you had to consume the food as
soon as it was still fresh since it didn't last very
long.

Fasting was the norm even in many "civilized" ancient nations. For instance, the Romans thought eating only one meal a day was better. They were preoccupied with digestion, and having many meals was seen as excess.

The Romans had a point from the standpoint of biological evolution.

Our brains function more quickly and with better attention when we speed, and our blood vessels expand and our muscles become more resistant to lactic acid buildup.

These reactions resulted in our prehistoric hunter-gatherer predecessors being better hunters, which seems simple when you think that the more hungry we are, the better we need to be at finding food.
On the other side, when we are overfed and continually eating, we develop extra weight and have slower movement and thought processes.

The Benefits of Intermittent Fasting

Intermittent fasting may have a number of advantages, including:

Weight reduction: By consuming fewer calories overall, intermittent fasting may aid in weight loss. Fasting forces your body to utilize its fat reserves as a source of energy, which might help you lose weight.

Increased insulin sensitivity: It has been shown that intermittent fasting increases insulin sensitivity, which may aid in controlling blood sugar levels. Blood pressure and cholesterol levels, two indicators of heart health, may benefit from improved insulin sensitivity as well.

Reduced inflammation: It has been shown that intermittent fasting lowers inflammatory levels in the body, which may provide protection against several illnesses.

Globally, chronic inflammatory diseases such as cancer, diabetes, obesity, and respiratory illnesses account for 3 out of 5 fatalities.

You could have less inflammation if you just ate one meal a day. By weakening pro-inflammatory cytokines in immune cells and enabling your gut lining to repair itself, fasting has been found to lessen inflammation.

Given that intestinal permeability, also known as leaky gut, enables plant toxins like lectins to enter the circulation, causing inflammation and exacerbating arthritis in numerous regions of the body, healing the gut lining may be crucial to managing inflammation.

According to research, mouse studies indicating that eating less often may improve longevity by as much as 80% can be attributed in large part to fasting's capacity to reduce inflammation.

The anti-inflammatory effects of both OMAD and a high-fat, low-carb ketogenic diet (speed keto) may be increased. Mitophagy, an anti-inflammatory, anti-aging mechanism, is fueled by ketones, the energy molecules generated during ketosis, which replenish your mitochondria and encourage new mitochondrial formation.

A Single Meal Per Day May Delay Aging

What happens if you just eat one meal every day? It's possible to feel younger and live longer.

According to one study, fasting for 24 hours increased levels of anti-aging chemicals, including human growth hormone (HGH), by 1300–2000%.

HGH is essential for the structure of skin, connective tissues, and muscle fibers.

According to 2021 research on fruit flies, which have DNA that is surprisingly similar to that of humans, a 20-hour fast routine increased longevity by 13% for men and 18% for women.

Researchers draw attention to the fact that the timing of the fast was crucial: only flies that fasted through the night and broke their fast around noon were found to live longer. There was no longer any gain in lifespan for the flies who fasted during the day and fed at night.

According to these studies, it may be necessary to have your one meal a day around midday in order to sync it with your circadian cycle and get its anti-aging advantages.

Alternate-day fasting has been shown in studies to lower indicators of aging-related frailty in older individuals.

One meal a day may be sufficient to support mental and emotional health.

One meal a day may boost the synthesis of neurochemicals and hormones linked to better mental and emotional wellbeing.

Your body creates a hormone called Brain-Derived Neurotrophic Factor when you are fasting (BDNF). John J. Ratey, a Harvard neuropsychiatrist, refers to it as "Miracle-Gro for the brain." Increased BDNF levels are linked to improved mood, improved cognition, and increased creativity.

According to other research, increased incidences of suicide due to depression are associated with low levels of BDNF.

Fasting's anti-inflammatory properties might benefit one's mental well-being and mood. Fasting is associated with increased levels of inflammation, and studies have shown that autophagy (the cellular rejuvenation that results from fasting) and depression both have anti-inflammatory effects.

Studies on mice demonstrate that a long-term intermittent fasting regimen significantly enhances cognition, learning, and memory.

Various studies on the impact of fasting on mental health were analyzed in 2021, and the results showed that it may alleviate stress, anxiety, and depression, particularly in non-pathological or moderate symptoms.

You avoid the post-lunch slump and the urge to boost energy with caffeinated beverages, which may worsen anxiety, when you eat meals centered on highly satiating keto foods that feed you throughout the day.

To further improve your mood, creativity, and mental clarity, combine eating just one meal each day with a short power nap in the middle of the afternoon.

One meal a day allows you more time and mental space.

Imagine a life if locating, cooking, and consuming food weren't continually stealing your wants, time, and logistical bandwidth. One of the most significant, but least discussed, effects of merely eating one meal every day is freedom.

OMAD may assist you in overcoming obstacles that prevent you from focusing on long-term objectives, enjoyable hobbies, self-improvement activities, and relationships that really nourish your heart and mind.

Other possible advantages: There may be further advantages to intermittent fasting, including enhanced mental performance and a lowered chance of developing certain illnesses, including cancer, Parkinson's disease, and Alzheimer's. To completely comprehend the consequences of intermittent fasting and the long-term safety of this eating pattern, further study is necessary.

In order to properly comprehend the consequences of intermittent fasting and the long-term safety of this eating pattern, it is vital to remember that further study is required. Before beginning any new eating pattern, it is wise to consult a healthcare provider.

Intermittent fasting could provide other advantages that have not yet been well investigated or comprehended. There is some evidence to indicate that intermittent fasting may enhance brain function, and some individuals who follow it claim to feel more energized and focused. Improvements in blood pressure and cholesterol levels, a decreased chance of developing specific illnesses including cancer and Alzheimer's disease, and increased immunological function are all other possible advantages of intermittent fasting that are currently being researched.

To completely comprehend the consequences of intermittent fasting and its long-term safety, it is crucial to keep in mind that additional study is required. Before beginning any new eating pattern, it is wise to consult a healthcare provider.

CHAPTER 2

Getting Started with OMAD Fasting

How to prepare for OMAD fasting/Tips for preparing for your first OMAD fast

Speak with a healthcare provider: Before beginning any new eating pattern, including OMAD fasting, it is always a good idea to see a healthcare provider. They can advise you on how to make sure you are obtaining adequate nutrients while observing this eating pattern and assist you in determining if OMAD fasting is appropriate for you.

Plan your meals: Planning your meals will assist you ensure that your one daily meal has the right amount of nutrients. Consider adding a range of fruits, vegetables, and whole grains, as well as nutrient-dense meals that are rich in protein, fiber, and healthy fats.

Maintaining enough hydration is crucial when on the OMAD diet. Make sure to drink enough of water, and think about include additional hydrating foods and drinks in your diet, including herbal tea or soups with broth.

Gradually adjust: If you are new to OMAD fasting, it could be beneficial to adjust to this eating pattern gradually. You may begin by experimenting with shorter fasting intervals, like the 16/8 technique, and then progressively lengthen your fasts over time.

When consuming foods that are part of the OMAD diet, it's critical to pay attention to your body's demands and how you feel. It can be important to modify your diet or take another dietary pattern into consideration if you feel you are not receiving enough nutrients or suffer any undesirable side effects.

Don't miss meals: It's critical to ensure that your one daily meal has adequate calories and nutrients. It might be challenging to follow your OMAD diet if you skip meals or don't eat enough, which can result in feelings of hunger and poor energy.

Eat slowly: Eating slowly may make you feel fuller after meals and may help you feel less hungry throughout the day.

Avoid distractions: Overeating may result from eating while multitasking, such as while watching TV or working on the internet. When you're eating, try to pay attention to your food and your hunger and fullness signs.

Sleep well: Getting adequate sleep is crucial for general health and may aid with weight control. Sleep for 7-9 hours every night.

Don't allow yourself get too hungry: If you experience extreme hunger while on the OMAD diet, you may need to modify your diet or think about switching to a new eating pattern. It's crucial to pay attention to your body's signals and make sure you're receiving the right amount of calories and nutrients.

How to set up your dining period

Here are some pointers for organizing your feeding window during an OMAD fast:

Pick a time that's convenient for you: Choose a time for your eating window that is convenient for you and enables you to have a healthy meal after taking your daily routine into account.

Eat slowly: Eating slowly may make you feel fuller after meals and may help you feel less hungry throughout the day.

Don't miss meals: It's critical to ensure that your one daily meal has adequate calories and nutrients. It might be challenging to follow your OMAD diet if you skip meals or don't eat enough, which can result in feelings of hunger and poor energy.

Eat a balanced meal: Include a mix of nutrient-dense foods, such as protein, fiber, and healthy fats, in your meal. Think about include a range of fresh produce, whole grains, and fruits.

Maintaining enough hydration is crucial when on the OMAD diet. Make sure to drink enough of water, and think about include additional hydrating foods and drinks in your diet, including herbal tea or soups with broth.

Ideas for Completing The Fast

Breaking your fast should always begin with a modest meal, and as you get acclimated to eating again, you may progressively increase your portion sizes. This may lessen bloating and uncomfortable symptoms.

Eat slowly: Eating slowly may make you feel fuller after meals and may help you feel less hungry throughout the day.

Pick nutrient-rich foods: When planning your meal, incorporate a range of nutrient-rich foods, including protein, fiber, and healthy fats. Think about including a range of fresh produce, whole grains, and fruits.

Maintaining enough hydration is crucial when on the OMAD diet. Make sure to drink enough of water, and think about include additional hydrating foods and drinks in your diet, including herbal tea or soups with broth.

Listen to your body's hunger and fullness signals and stop eating when you are content rather than when you are stuffed: It is crucial to pay attention to your body's hunger and fullness signs. This may encourage weight reduction and stop overeating.

Success strategies for the OMAD fast

Typical Errors to Prevent

Not receiving enough nutrients: Getting all the nutrients you need in a single regular meal might be difficult. Make sure to choose meals that are high in nutrients and pay attention to what your body requires.

Overeating: Pay attention to your hunger and fullness signals and stop eating when you are satisfied rather than when you are stuffed. The potential advantages of OMAD fasting may be defeated by overeating and result in weight gain.

Not drinking enough water: When following the OMAD diet, drinking enough water is crucial. Make sure to drink enough of water, and think about include additional hydrating foods and drinks in your diet, including herbal tea or soups with broth.

Meal skipping: It's critical to ensure that your one daily meal has adequate calories and minerals. It might be challenging to follow your OMAD diet if you skip meals or don't eat enough, which can result in feelings of hunger and poor energy.

being too rigid: It's crucial to be adaptable and mindful of your body's demands. Making changes or thinking about switching to a new eating pattern may be essential if you are having trouble sticking to your OMAD diet.

Lack of sleep: Getting adequate sleep is essential for good health and may also aid with weight control. Sleep for 7-9 hours every night.

Overeating may result from eating while preoccupied, such as while watching television or using a computer. When you're eating, try to pay attention to your food and your hunger and fullness signs.

Being inconsistent: In order to see benefits, it's critical to follow your OMAD fasting plan consistently. To create a habit, try to adhere to the same eating window each day.

being impatient: OMAD fasting outcomes might take time to manifest. Being patient and giving oneself time to become used to this food pattern is crucial.

Not seeking assistance: While adhering to an OMAD diet, it may be beneficial to seek support from friends, family, or a medical professional.

You may be motivated and on track as a result of this.

CHAPTER 3

Meal Planning and Preparation

The importance of nutrient-dense foods during OMAD fasting.

The significance of consuming nutrient-dense meals when on an OMAD fast
To ensure that you are obtaining enough nutrients to suit your body's demands while on an OMAD fast, it is crucial to pick nutrient-dense meals. Foods that are abundant in nutrients yet low in calories are said to be nutrient-dense. They are a crucial component of a balanced diet and may guard against nutritional shortages.

Foods that are high in nutrients include the following:

Fruits and vegetables: These are low in calories and rich in vitamins, minerals, and fiber.

Examples of lean protein sources include chicken, fish, beans, and tofu. Protein may help you feel full and is necessary for muscle growth and maintenance.

Examples of good fats include olive oil, almonds, and avocados. Healthy fats may keep you feeling full and are beneficial for your heart.

Whole grains: Quinoa, oats, and brown rice are a few examples. Because they are rich in fiber, whole grains may aid in regulating digestion and keeping you full.

While following an OMAD diet, you may help to ensure that you are obtaining enough nutrients to suit your body's requirements by adding a range of nutrient-dense foods in your daily meals.

Deficiencies in certain nutrients: It's critical to ensure that you are consuming enough nutrients to support your body's demands while on the OMAD diet. You may be at risk for nutritional deficiencies if you do not consume enough nutrients, which might have a severe impact on your health.

Weight reduction: By supplying your body with the nutrients it needs while limiting calorie consumption, choosing nutrient-dense meals may encourage weight loss.

Foods that are rich in nutrients and fiber might help you feel full and satisfied for longer. This is particularly crucial if you're on the OMAD diet since you'll be consuming all of your daily caloric intake at once.

Foods high in nutrients may assist provide your body the energy it needs to operate efficiently. This is crucial if you're on the OMAD diet since you can be fasting for a long time.

While adhering to an OMAD diet, you may help to ensure that you are getting enough nutrients to satisfy your body's demands by selecting nutrient-dense foods. A healthcare expert should always be consulted for advice on how to make sure you are consuming enough nutrients to fulfill your specific needs.

Grass-fed and pasture-raised ruminant meats as well as conventional meat
Good fats from entire foods
complete organ meats
fatty fish such as sardines, mackerel, and wild salmon
nutrient-dense seafood such as salmon roe, oysters, shrimp, and mussels
nourishing drinks like keto butter coffee and other low-carb keto drinks for intermittent fasting
Eggs
Full-fat dairy products, such as cheese, yogurt, and cream for those who can consume them

It's also crucial to adjust your OMAD macros and calories such that you consume 1500–2000 calories daily.

The goal of OMAD is not to deprive yourself of food and starve yourself. In fact, it's preferable to see weight reduction as a positive byproduct of a far more comprehensive health and wellness makeover rather than the intended goal.

Here are Samples Meal Plans for OMAD

1 Grilled chicken breast with roasted vegetables and quinoa

2 Baked salmon with steamed broccoli and brown rice

3 Turkey and vegetable stir-fry with brown rice

4 Black bean and vegetable burrito with avocado and brown rice

5 Vegetable and tofu curry with quinoa

6 Grilled shrimp with roasted sweet potatoes and asparagus

7 Veggie burger with roasted potatoes and Brussels sprouts

8 Baked chicken with roasted root vegetables and wild rice

9 Grilled salmon with roasted Brussels sprouts and sweet potatoes

10 Beef and broccoli stir-fry with brown rice

11 Black bean and vegetable quesadilla with avocado and brown rice

12 Grilled chicken with roasted zucchini and quinoa

13 Grilled shrimp with steamed broccoli and brown rice

14 Baked salmon with roasted asparagus and sweet potatoes

15 Grilled chicken with roasted vegetables and brown rice

16 Tofu and vegetable stir-fry with quinoa

17 Grilled salmon with roasted Brussels sprouts and brown rice

18 Beef and broccoli with brown rice
Veggie burger with roasted sweet potatoes and asparagus

19 Grilled chicken with roasted zucchini and quinoa

20 Grilled shrimp with roasted root vegetables and wild rice

21 Baked salmon with steamed broccoli and brown rice

23. Black bean and vegetable enchiladas with avocado and brown rice

24 Grilled chicken with roasted asparagus and sweet potatoes

25 Tofu and vegetable curry with quinoa

26 Grilled shrimp with roasted Brussels sprouts and sweet potatoes

27 Baked salmon with roasted root vegetables and wild rice

28 Veggie burger with roasted zucchini and quinoa

29 Grilled chicken with steamed broccoli and brown rice

30 Beef and broccoli with brown rice and roasted vegetables.

31 Grilled chicken with roasted sweet potatoes and asparagus

32 Tofu and vegetable stir-fry with brown rice

33 Grilled salmon with roasted root vegetables and wild rice

34 Veggie burger with roasted Brussels sprouts and sweet potatoes

35 Grilled chicken with steamed broccoli and brown rice

36 Baked salmon with roasted zucchini and quinoa

37 Black bean and vegetable burrito with avocado and brown rice

38 Grilled shrimp with roasted asparagus and sweet potatoes

39 Tofu and vegetable curry with quinoa

40 Grilled chicken with roasted root vegetables and wild rice

41 Grilled salmon with steamed broccoli and brown rice

42 Beef and broccoli with brown rice and roasted vegetables

43 Veggie burger with roasted zucchini and quinoa

44 Grilled chicken with roasted Brussels sprouts and sweet potatoes

45 Grilled shrimp with roasted root vegetables and wild rice

46 Baked salmon with steamed broccoli and brown rice

47 Black bean and vegetable enchiladas with avocado and brown rice

48 Grilled chicken with roasted asparagus and sweet potatoes

49 Grilled salmon with roasted Brussels sprouts and brown rice

50 Beef and broccoli with brown rice
Veggie burger with roasted root vegetables and wild rice

Ideas for High-Protein, Low-Carb Meals

1 Grilled chicken with roasted vegetables
2 Baked salmon with steamed broccoli

3 Turkey and vegetable stir-fry

4 Grilled shrimp with roasted sweet   potatoes

5 Grilled chicken with roasted asparagus

7 Beef and broccoli stir-fry

8 Grilled salmon with roasted Brussels sprouts

9 Baked chicken with roasted root vegetables

10 Grilled shrimp with steamed broccoli

11 Grilled chicken with roasted zucchini

12 Tofu and vegetable stir-fry

13 Grilled salmon with roasted asparagus

14 Grilled chicken with roasted root vegetables

15 Beef and broccoli with roasted vegetables

16 Grilled shrimp with roasted Brussels sprouts

17 Baked salmon with steamed broccoli

18 Grilled chicken with roasted zucchini

19 Tofu and vegetable curry

20 Grilled salmon with roasted root vegetables

21 Grilled chicken with roasted asparagus

22 Grilled shrimp with roasted sweet potatoes

23 Baked salmon with roasted Brussels sprouts

24 Grilled chicken with roasted root vegetables

25 Beef and broccoli with roasted vegetables

26 Grilled shrimp with steamed broccoli

27 Grilled chicken with roasted zucchini

28 Tofu and vegetable stir-fry

29 Grilled salmon with roasted asparagus

30 Grilled chicken with roasted root vegetables

Snack Options for Between Meals

1 Hard-boiled eggs

2 Greek yogurt with berries

3 Nuts and seeds

4 Hummus with vegetables

5 Apple slices with nut butter

6 Edamame

7 Cottage cheese with fruit

8 Turkey slices with avocado

9 Roasted chickpeas

10 Protein smoothie

11 Trail mix

12 Protein bar

13 Carrot sticks with hummus

14 Olives

15 Boiled eggs with avocado
16 Cucumber slices with peanut butter
17 Cheese sticks
18 Protein balls
19 Rice cakes with almond butter
20 Beef jerky

CHAPTER 4

Managing Hunger and Cravings

Strategies for managing hunger during OMAD fasting

Eat a nutrient-dense meal: Include a range of nutrient-dense meals, such as protein, fiber, and healthy fats, in your daily meal. You may continue to feel content and full as a result.

Be sure to stay hydrated by drinking plenty of water. This will assist to curb your appetite. Water should be consumed in large amounts throughout the day.

Add more healthy fats to your diet: Eating more healthy fats might help you feel full and pleased. Avocados, almonds, and olive oil are all excellent sources of healthful fats.

Remain active: Regular physical exercise might assist to increase metabolism and lessen feelings of hunger.

Find good coping mechanisms for stress since it might make you feel hungry. Find healthy coping mechanisms for stress, such as meditation, exercise, or talking to a friend or therapist.

Snacking on high-protein, low-calorie meals might help you feel full and pleased without adding too many calories to your diet. Greek yogurt, almonds, seeds, and hard-boiled eggs are a few examples.

Don't miss meals: Even though OMAD fasting only calls for one meal each day, it's still crucial to receive the right amount of nutrients for your body. Skipping meals might make you feel hungry and is not likely to be sustainable over time.

Eat mindfully: Being aware of your hunger and fullness signals may help you better understand your body's demands and regulate your appetite. Avoid distractions when you're eating and try to concentrate on your meal.

Consume more fiber-rich foods to help you feel fuller and more content. Fruits and vegetables, whole grains, and legumes are among examples.

How to Handle Cravings and Food Temptations

Although resisting food temptations and satisfying cravings might be difficult, doing so is crucial to maintaining a balanced diet and way of life. Here are a few more techniques that might be useful:

In advance: Having a plan in place might lessen the likelihood of giving in to food cravings.

Make a list of the foods you need and stick to it. You should also have some healthy snack alternatives on available.

Consume mindfully: Eating while paying attention to your hunger and fullness signals may help to curb cravings and increase your awareness of the foods you choose to eat. Avoid distractions when you're eating and try to concentrate on your meal.

Keep hydrated: Drinking a lot of water will help you feel full and cut down on cravings. Always carry a water bottle with you and make an effort to consume at least 8 glasses of water each day.

Discover good coping mechanisms for stress since it might lead to cravings. Find healthy coping mechanisms for stress, such as meditation, exercise, or talking to a friend or therapist.

When attempting to control cravings and food temptations, seeking assistance from friends, family, or a healthcare provider may be beneficial. This might give you a feeling of responsibility and keep you motivated.

Use moderation while eating since overeating may lead to cravings and food temptations. Use smaller dishes and bowls and measure out portions of food to practice portion management. This may lessen the likelihood of overeating and perhaps lessen cravings.

Consume adequate protein since it promotes fullness and may lessen cravings. Eat meals high in protein, such as lean meats, eggs, almonds, and beans.

Find healthy substitutes: If you have a hankering for a certain meal, attempt to find a healthy substitute that will satisfy the need. You may, for instance, eat a piece of fruit or a tiny portion of dark chocolate if you are desiring something sweet.

When a hunger comes, attempt to divert your attention with anything else. This may be chatting to a buddy, taking a stroll, or reading a book.

CHAPTER 5

Staying Active and Maintaining Energy

The Role of Exercise During OMAD Fasting

Increasing energy: Exercise on a regular basis may assist to enhance general fitness and raise energy levels.

Supporting weight control: A balanced diet and exercise may assist weight management.

Health advantages of exercise include strengthening bones and muscles, lowering the chance of developing certain chronic conditions, and improving cardiovascular health.

Exercise has been demonstrated to assist in lowering stress levels and elevating mood.

Enhancing sleep: Exercise may assist to enhance the amount and quality of sleep.

Managing hunger: Exercise may aid in reducing hunger sensations and may make it simpler to maintain an OMAD fasting schedule.

Exercise has been demonstrated to increase cognitive function and mental clarity, improving concentration and clarity of thought. This may aid to increase attention and productivity while engaging in an OMAD fasting regimen.

Relaxation: Exercise may aid in promoting relaxation and lowering tension and anxiety levels. When engaging in OMAD fasting, this might be advantageous since it could enhance general health.

Digestive system stimulation and improvement may be achieved via exercise. When adhering to an OMAD fasting regimen, this might be useful since it could enhance the absorption of nutrients from the day meal.

Ideas for Low-intensity Workouts During Fasting Periods

Here are some suggestions for low-intensity exercises you may do while adhering to an OMAD intermittent fasting schedule:

Walking is a low-impact, convenient exercise that you can perform anywhere. Anyone searching for a low-intensity workout or someone new to exercising might consider it.

Yoga: Yoga is a mind-body workout with little impact that may be performed at home or in a studio. Flexibility, strength, and balance may all be enhanced.

Pilates: Pilates is a low-impact workout that emphasizes stability and core strength. It may be performed with tools or a mat in a studio or at home.

Swimming: Swimming may be done in a pool and is a low-impact workout. It is a fantastic alternative for those who have joint problems or want a low-impact training.

Tai chi: Slow, controlled motions are used in this low-impact, mind-body exercise. It may be performed at home or in a studio and might enhance flexibility and balance.

Low-impact exercise that may be performed both outdoors and on a stationary bike is biking. Lower body strength and cardiovascular fitness may also benefit from it.

Resistance band exercises: Resistance band exercises are a low-impact approach to increase muscular tone and strength. Resistance bands may be used to perform them in a studio or at home.

Hiking is a low-impact outdoor exercise that may assist to increase lower body strength and cardiovascular fitness.

Aquatic exercise: Water aerobics is a low-impact exercise that may be performed in a pool. Lower body strength and cardiovascular fitness may also benefit from it.

Elliptical machine: You may use the elliptical machine at home or at the gym to do low-impact cardiovascular exercises. Lower body strength and cardiovascular fitness may also benefit from it.

CHAPTER 6

OMAD Fasting for Specific Health Goals

Weight loss with OMAD fasting

OMAD fasting may promote weight reduction via a number of different ways, including the following:
Calorie reduction: By just eating one meal each day, you may unintentionally lower your calorie intake. Over time, this might result in weight loss.
Intermittent fasting may boost the release of fatty acids from adipose tissue, which may be utilized as an energy source, according to some study. Losing weight might be facilitated by this.

Increased insulin sensitivity: It has been shown that intermittent fasting increases insulin sensitivity, which may aid in weight control.

Hormone balance is improved by intermittent fasting, which may aid in weight control by improving the balance of specific hormones including ghrelin and leptin.

Increased physical activity: Some individuals who practice OMAD fasting may discover that it gives them more energy for exercise, which may aid in weight reduction.

Improved digestion: The OMAD diet may help with digestion and nutrition absorption, which may encourage weight reduction.

Improving insulin sensitivity and blood sugar control with OMAD fasting

Potential ways through which OMAD fasting may enhance insulin sensitivity and blood sugar regulation include the following:

Calorie reduction: By eating just one meal each day, you may naturally lower your calorie intake, which over time may increase your body's sensitivity to insulin and ability to regulate your blood sugar levels.

Intermittent fasting may boost the release of fatty acids from adipose tissue, which may be utilized as an energy source, according to some study. This could enhance blood sugar regulation and insulin sensitivity.

Hormone balance is improved by intermittent fasting, which may aid in blood sugar regulation by improving the balance of specific hormones including ghrelin and leptin.

Reduced inflammation: According to some study, intermittent fasting may lessen the body's inflammatory response, which might enhance insulin sensitivity and blood sugar regulation.

Increased physical activity: Some individuals who follow an OMAD fasting schedule may discover that it gives them more energy for exercise, which may help regulate blood sugar levels.

Improved absorption of nutrients from food: OMAD fasting may result in improved digestion and absorption of nutrients, which may help blood sugar regulation.

CHAPTER 7

Frequently Asked Questions about OMAD Fasting

Is OMAD Fasting Safe for Everyone?

Potential ways through which OMAD fasting may enhance insulin sensitivity and blood sugar regulation include the following:

Calorie reduction: By eating just one meal each day, you may naturally lower your calorie intake, which over time may increase your body's sensitivity to insulin and ability to regulate your blood sugar levels.

Intermittent fasting may boost the release of fatty acids from adipose tissue, which may be utilized as an energy source, according to some study. This could enhance blood sugar regulation and insulin sensitivity.

Hormone balance is improved by intermittent fasting, which may aid in blood sugar regulation by improving the balance of specific hormones including ghrelin and leptin.

Reduced inflammation: According to some study, intermittent fasting may lessen the body's inflammatory response, which might enhance insulin sensitivity and blood sugar regulation.

Increased physical activity: Some individuals who follow an OMAD fasting schedule may discover that it gives them more energy for exercise, which may help regulate blood sugar levels.

Improved absorption of nutrients from food: OMAD fasting may result in improved digestion and absorption of nutrients, which may help blood sugar regulation.

How long Should I Practice OMAD Fasting?

Before beginning any new fitness or nutritional program, including OMAD fasting, it is always a good idea to speak with a healthcare provider. They may assist in assessing your particular requirements and provide advice on how long practicing OMAD fasting is suitable and safe.

It is generally not advised to engage in OMAD for a lengthy period of time. Instead than being a long-term eating strategy, intermittent fasting should be a transient dietary trend. To make sure that you are receiving all the nutrients your body needs to operate effectively, it is crucial to maintain a diverse and balanced diet.

Setting a time limit for your fast, such as one week or one month, then reevaluating your success and general wellbeing at the conclusion of that period may be useful if you're thinking of engaging in OMAD fasting. By doing this, you can make sure that you aren't engaging in OMAD fasting for a lengthy amount of time and that your general health and wellbeing are a top priority.

Own objectives: Take into account how long it can take you to accomplish your personal objectives. For instance, if losing weight is your aim, you can opt to follow OMAD fasting for a certain length of time and then reevaluate your results.

general well-being and health: While engaging in OMAD fasting, keep an eye on your general health and wellbeing. It could be time to quit engaging in OMAD fasting if you experience any unfavorable alterations, such as less energy, trouble focusing, or vitamin deficits.

Consumption of nutrients: To make sure you are receiving all the nutrients your body requires, eat a range of nutrient-dense meals in each daily meal. It could be time to discontinue OMAD fasting if you can't get all the nutrients you need.

Sustainability: Think about if OMAD fasting is a long-term sustainable eating pattern for you. It may not be a sustainable choice for you if you have trouble sticking to the routine or if it is not pleasurable for you.

CHAPTER 8

Tips for Maintaining your OMAD Fasting Practice

The following advice will help you continue your OMAD (One Meal a Day) fasting routine:

In advance: Making a schedule for your meals and snacks will help you stay on track with your OMAD fasting schedule and ensuring that you have the things you need on hand.

Tracking your progress may help you remain on track and recognize the improvement you are making. Some ways to do this include maintaining a food journal or using a fitness app. Keep yourself hydrated: Drinking enough of water might help you feel full and less hungry. Water should be consumed in large amounts throughout the day.

Get adequate sleep: Getting enough sleep is crucial for general health and may aid with blood sugar regulation. Sleep for 7-9 hours every night.

Exercise regularly: Regular exercise may assist to increase insulin sensitivity and blood sugar regulation. Think about include exercises like walking, jogging, cycling, or strength training in your daily routine.

You may be able to sustain your OMAD fasting routine and accomplish your objectives by paying attention to these suggestions. To get advice on how to improve general health and wellbeing, don't forget to speak with a healthcare expert.

Find a support network: Having a network of people to turn to for encouragement and accountability, such as a friend or family member who also engages in OMAD fasting or a medical expert, may be helpful.

Be present throughout mealtimes. Focus on eating slowly and deliberately. Take your time. This may assist you in feeling full and preventing overeating.

Find techniques to cope with stress: Maintaining general health and wellbeing may require effective stress management. Think about introducing stress-reduction practices like yoga or meditation into your daily routine.

Be adaptable: It's OK to periodically stray from your OMAD fasting schedule, but be sure to get back on track as soon as you can. Don't let failures halt your advancement.

Recap of the benefits of OMAD fasting

The possible advantages of an OMAD (One Meal a Day) fast are listed as follows:
Weight loss: According to some study, OMAD fasting may help people lose weight by lowering calorie intake and boosting fat burning.

Improved insulin sensitivity and blood sugar regulation: By consuming fewer calories, enhancing fat burning, and balancing hormones, OMAD fasting may enhance insulin sensitivity and blood sugar regulation.

Increased physical activity: Some individuals who practice OMAD fasting may discover that it gives them more energy for exercise, which may benefit their general health and wellbeing. Hormone balance may be improved by OMAD fasting, which may boost general health and wellbeing by balancing key hormones like ghrelin and leptin.
Reduced inflammation: According to some study, OMAD fasting may lower the body's inflammatory response, which is beneficial for general health and wellbeing.

CONCLUSION

In conclusion, OMAD (One Meal a Day) fasting is a type of intermittent fasting that involves eating just one meal per day. This dietary pattern has the potential to provide a number of benefits, including weight loss, improved insulin sensitivity and blood sugar control, increased physical activity, improved hormone balance, and reduced inflammation.

However, it is important to note that the effects of OMAD fasting may vary, and more research is needed to fully understand the mechanisms involved. It is always a good idea to consult a healthcare professional before starting any new dietary or exercise routine, including OMAD fasting. They can help to evaluate your individual needs and provide guidance on whether OMAD fasting is appropriate for you.

If you choose to incorporate OMAD fasting into your routine, it is important to prioritize overall health and well-being and to have a varied and balanced diet. Make sure to include a variety of nutrient-dense foods in your daily meal to ensure that you are getting all the nutrients your body needs. In addition, consider incorporating strategies such as planning ahead, staying hydrated, getting enough sleep, and engaging in physical activity to help you maintain your OMAD fasting practice.

By following these tips and consulting a healthcare professional, you can optimize your OMAD fasting practice and achieve your health and wellness goals. Remember to listen to your body and prioritize overall health and well-being.

www.ingramcontent.com/pod-product-compliance
Lightning Source LLC
LaVergne TN
LVHW020055060225
803089LV00029B/1255